HORMONAL BALANCE

7 Steps to Wellness

CRISTINA ABATE

Disclaimer

The information is of a general nature and does not take into account your personal situation. The information presented is for educational purposes only. The author will not bear any responsibility or liability for any action taken by any person, persons or organization on the purported basis of the information contained in this book and any supporting material. References to other information, websites or events should not be understood as an endorsement of such information, website or events. Every effort has been made to ensure that this book is free from errors or omissions. However, the author shall not accept responsibility for injury, loss or damage occasioned to any person acting or refraining from action as a result of material in this book whether or not such injury, loss or damage is in any way due to any negligent act or omission, breach of duty or default on the part of the author.

CONTENTS

INTRODUCTION

I want to thank you and congratulate you for buying this book, "**Hormonal Balance**".

This book contains proven steps and strategies on how to keep your hormones balanced.

It also includes some recipes for healthy herbal teas and homemade house cleaners to help lower toxins in your home that can effect or cause hormonal imbalance.

There are tips on what to include in your diet that will help to provide your body with the building blocks it needs to keep your hormones in a healthy balanced state.

This book is a quick read and is packed with valuable information on the topic of hormones from beginning to end.

I hope you take the information provided in my book and put it to good use. It will help you build a healthy way of life and once you do that your hormones will start to balance out in a healthy manner leaving you feeling energized and full of life!

Thanks again for purchasing this book, I hope you enjoy it!

WHAT ARE HORMONES?

Hormones are the chemical messengers of your body. They travel in your blood stream in order to reach various organs and tissues in your body. They work over time at a slow rate affecting many different processes, including:

- Mood
- Reproduction
- Sexual function
- Metabolism - this is how your body gets energy from the foods you consume
- Growth development

Hormones are made from a special group of cells called Endocrine glands. The major endocrine glands are the adrenal glands, thyroid, thymus, pineal, pancreas, and pituitary. Women produce hormones in their ovaries and men produce them in their testes.

Good fats and cholesterol produce hormones, so if you are lacking these important dietary factors this can cause hormone problems to develop because the body is unable to make the hormones because it is missing the building blocks it needs to make them.

Problems also occur when toxins containing chemicals that either mimics the hormones or the building blocks needed to make them can be very problematic. The body could end up trying to create the hormones using the wrong building blocks which could result in mutant estrogen.

We probably will never totally understand all the complexities of the endocrine system but there are some basic things that you can do in order to boost your body's natural ability to create and balance hormones.

People may not be aware of just how big an effect hormones and gut bacteria have on our overall health. Even if you are doing well in other areas such as eating a healthy diet, taking supplements etc. These two factors can destroy your health if they are not functioning properly.

It is believed by many that by fixing problems with hormones and gut bacteria can help to boost your health in other areas. Studies have shown that certain hormone reactions can heal brain trauma.

Hormones have a very real power that can affect many different things in the body from bowel health, mood, and weight. I am sure if you asked any woman that is or was pregnant what kind of changes they experienced in their bodies while being pregnant they will have a story to share with you. Pregnancy is a common time in which a woman's hormones could be out of balance.

You could be suffering from hormone imbalance if you have symptoms such as: skin issues, weight gain, fatigue, and weight around your middle, PMS, trouble sleeping, endometriosis, infertility, PCOS or other issues.

STEP 1

AVOID TOXINS

You can find toxins in plastics, pesticides, household chemicals, your mattress may even contain hormone disrupting chemicals these mimic hormones in the body which keep the body from producing real hormones. Hormonal birth control can do the same thing.

Avoiding toxins is very important even more so if you are trying to get pregnant and especially if you have a hormone imbalance. When you are cooking use non-coated metal pans or glass. Do not use non-stick or Teflon! Try not to store or heat your foods in plastic. Do not use chemical cleaners or pesticides. When shopping for foods go for organic produce and meat whenever you can.

Recipe for All-Purpose Natural Cleaner:

Ingredients:
- 1 tsp. Of borax
- ½ tsp. Of washing soda
- 1 tsp. Of liquid castille soap
- essential oils as preferred - I use 4 drops of lemon, 4 drops of lavender and 10 drops of Orange

Instructions:

3

1. Add 2 cups of warm water, distilled is the best, water that has been boiled will work. I use as a bathroom cleaner, kitchen cleaner, and floor pre-treater.

.

STEP 2

REDUCING TOXINS IN YOUR HOME

The air within our homes is generally more polluted than the air outside. So to help filter out harmful toxins in our home air here is a list of 10 house plants that can help you make the air quality in your home healthier and achieving it in a natural way. This is a fun green way to help fight against toxins that can lead to hormonal imbalances.

10 House plants that will help to improve air quality

1. **Aloe (Aloe Vera)**. This is a great plant that loves sunlight is succulent and will help to clear formaldehyde and benzene, which are byproducts of paints, chemical based cleaners, and more. This will work great in a sunny kitchen window not only will it clean the air but the gel found in the leaves of the plant can help to heal cuts and burns.

2. **Spider Plant**. The spider plant is quite a resilient plant it will battle benzene, formaldehyde, carbon monoxide and xylene, a solvent used in leather, printing and rubber industries. It is also known as a safe house plants if you have pets.

3. **Gerber Daisy**. This is a lovely bright flowered plant that can remove trichloroethylene, which could enter your home through your dry cleaning. It helps filter out benzene that comes with inks. This is a good plant to add to your laundry room or bedroom in a spot with lots of light.

4. Snake Plant. This plant is also known as mother-in-law's tongue, this is one of the best plants for filtering out formaldehyde, which is commonly found in toilet paper, cleaning products, and personal care products. This would thrive in your bathroom and provide you with a great filter of air pollutants.

5. Golden pothos. This is a great powerful plant for fighting against formaldehyde; it is a fast-growing vine will create a lovely hanging form in your home. A good place to put one is in your garage as there is a lot of formaldehyde there is the car exhaust if filled with it.

6. Chrysanthemum. This is a plant that not only gives you a lovely range of colorful flowers but it will help to filter out benzene which is commonly found in plastics, paint, and glue. Make sure to keep it in a place where it would get direct sunlight.

7. Red-edged dracaena. The red edges give a wonderful bit of color; this shrub can grow to your ceiling. It will help to remove trichloroethylene and formaldehyde that is introduced into your home through the uses of varnish, gasoline and lacquers.

8. Weeping Figs. This plant can help to filter out pollutants that are found in carpeting and furniture such as formaldehyde, benzene and trichloroethylene.

9. Azalea this beautiful shrub will help to fight against formaldehyde that comes from plywood, or foam insulation. They prefer a cool area they would be good to have in the basement.

10. English Ivy. This great plant is known to remove formaldehyde and also airborne fecal-matter particles.

Other Natural Air Cleaners:

One way to help in avoiding hormonal imbalance triggered by toxins is by trying to reduce chemical exposure any way you can such as by using house plants as I mentioned in the previous and here is a couple more natural air cleaners I would suggest trying.

Bamboo Charcoal
You can use "Moso air purifying bags that are filled with bamboo charcoal and put into linen bags. The bamboo charcoal will help to dehumidify the air and absorb unpleasant odors. These will work great in removing toxins

and odors from your homes air. The bamboo charcoal has a porous structure with a high density that is great at removing harmful pollutants, bacteria, and allergens from the air and also removes moisture preventing mold and mildew by trapping the moisture within each pore. The Moso air purifying bag has been scientifically tested and proven to reduce the amount of such toxins as: formaldehyde, chloroform gases that are emitted daily from items such as paint, furniture, carpets, chemical cleaners, plastics, and rubbers, benzene and ammonia. The bags are toxin free so they are safe to use around your pets and children. You can rejuvenate the charcoal bags by placing them in sunlight for up to two years. At that point you can take the charcoal and pour it onto your soil surrounding your houseplants to fertilize and help them in retaining moisture. I would suggest putting a Moso bag in each room of your house.

Salt Lamps

These are another great natural way to clean your indoor air supply. They are made from Himalayan salt crystals they release negative ions into your house air supply this helps to clean the air. They are a lovely light source. It is also a good air purifier when it is lit the negative ions that it emits fight against positively charged particles that can cause you to feel sluggish and stuffy. When the salt crystal is lit it clears the air of allergens, pet dander, pollens, and other air pollutants in a natural way.

People with asthma often find it helpful in reducing their symptoms as it helps to dilute odors so that you can breathe easier. Keep the lamp lit as long as you like to maintain this purifying effect. These lamps can make great reading lamps and the orange natural glow doesn't have a negative effect on your sleep hormones like blue lights or fluorescent lights do. Instead it is a very relaxing and natural light source.

Beeswax Candles

These candles can burn with almost no smoke or scent and they will clean the air when they release ions into the air. These negative ions that the beeswax candles release will help to remove toxins from your home air.

STEP 3

AVOID HIGH OMEGA-6 POLYUNSATURATED FATS

Vegetable oils contain very high levels of polyunsaturated fats.

Our bodies need fat for rebuilding cells and hormone production but our bodies have to use the building blocks that we give it.

Instead of giving our bodies the ratios they need we end up giving them loads of polyunsaturated fats. Our bodies then try and incorporate these fats into our cells during cell repair and cell creation.

The big problem here is that polyunsaturated fats are highly unstable and tend to oxidize easily in the body if they haven't already done this while sitting on a grocery shelf while getting exposure to sunlight. These oxidized fats then cause mutation in the cells and inflammation.

The arteries can become clogged when the arterial cells develop inflammation due to these mutations.

These fats can also cause skin cancer if they are incorporated into skin cells.

These unhealthy fats can also cause problems that can result in you having hormone imbalance.

Oils and Fats That You Should Avoid:

- Any fake butter or vegetable oils products
- Shortening
- Margarine
- Grape seed oil
- Cottonseed oil
- Safflower oil
- Sunflower oil
- Peanut oil
- Soybean oil
- Canola oil

There is no nutritional value in these products you can find healthy fats in higher amounts and in better ratios in many other types of fats.

Healthy Fats to Use:

Coconut Oil: This is filled with Chain fatty acids and Lauric acid this is a great source for saturated fats. Coconut oil does not oxidize easily and is a good choice in baking and cooking.

Meats: Grass fed meats has a higher nutrient level with healthy forms of saturated fats and omega-3s. Try and consume these types of meat.

Butter: This is an excellent source of fat soluble vitamins, and saturated fat as well as other nutrients.

Avocado Oil: This is a good source of monounsaturated fats is good for using with salads.

Palm Oil: This is high in saturated fat.

Olive Oil: This is high in monounsaturated fats and low in polyunsaturated fats it really isn't good for cooking with as high temperatures can make it susceptible to oxidation.

Organic Cream: This is a good source of saturated fat; organic heavy cream is basically liquid butter.

Eggs: Eggs are loaded with healthy fats and cholesterol as well as vitamins. Try and eat organic eggs.

Fish: Fish has high Omega-3 fatty acids and can help to balance Omega-3 and Omega-6 levels in the body. Wild caught best.

.

STEP 4

LIMIT CAFFEINE CONSUMPTION

Like most people I love drinking coffee but too much caffeine can really cause problems for your endocrine system, especially if there are other hormone stressors involved such as the presence of toxins, pregnancy, or beneficial fat imbalance or stress.

If you know that you drink way too much coffee perhaps it is time to look at replacing it with another healthier beverage such as herbal teas.

If you do not want to try giving up your coffee then try and add 1 tablespoon of coconut oil to each cup and blend it in the blender to emulsify. It will be like having a latte but with healthy fats!

Creamy Delicious & Nutritionally Packed Coffee Recipe

Ingredients:
- 1 cup of organic fresh made coffee or herbal coffee
- 1 tablespoon of coconut oil or more I use 3
- 1 teaspoon of organic butter
- ¼ teaspoon of vanilla
- Optional some Stevia natural sweetener to taste

Herbal Tea Recipes with Health Benefits

Stomach Soother: This is a good tea if you have stomach aches or have digestive troubles it is a very calming tea.
Ingredients:

- 2 teaspoons of mint leaf
- ½ teaspoon of fennel seeds
- Pinch of dried ginger (optional)
- Pour a cup of boiling water over it and steep for 5 minutes then consume.

Chai Tea: This is a great tea to have at night time.
Ingredients:

- 4 cups of coconut milk
- 8 tea bags of herbal tea I use Tetley's Chai tea bags
- 1-2 teaspoons of Stevia
- About 7 fresh slices of ginger root
- 6 cinnamon sticks
- 8 whole cloves
- 1 teaspoon of vanilla

Instructions:
Put water in a crock pot and add herbs and spices
Cook on high for about 2 hours or keep on low overnight. Add milk or coconut milk stir until well blended.
You can serve plain or top with real whipped cream sprinkled with cinnamon. You can also chill it and serve cold just blend it with some ice and 2 tablespoons of coconut oil.
Now sit back and enjoy!

Lavender Tea: I love the smell of lavender essential oil but Lavender is too strong to use alone in tea.
Ingredients:
½ cup of mint leaf
2 tablespoons of Stevia
2 tablespoons of Dried Lavender

Instructions:
Mix these entire ingredients together blend well then store in an air-tight container. Use 1-2 teaspoons per cup of water to make a hot or iced tea.

Raspberry Leaf Tea: This is a highly nutritious tea and is very beneficial for women as it helps in balancing hormones and is very good for the skin.

It is also a good source of Potassium, Magnesium, and B-Vitamins which is good to drink during pregnancy as it can help to strengthen the uterus.

STEP 5

SUPPLEMENTING WISELY

To help keep your hormones balanced it is a good idea to take some basic supplements that specifically help to support hormone balance.

Below are specific supplements that will help support hormone balance.

Gelatin: This is a great source of calcium, magnesium, and phosphate. It helps to support hormone production as well as helps in soothing inflammation especially in joints and digestive health.

Fermented Cod Liver Oil: This is a great source for necessary building blocks for hormone production including Vitamins A, D and K. It is also a great source for beneficial fats and Omega-3s.

Vitamin D: This is a pre-hormone that is supportive of hormone function. The best way to get Vitamin D is from the sun or from a D3 supplement.

Magnesium: Hundreds of reactions in the body are supported by Magnesium it often contributes to better sleep which is great for hormones. You can get it in several forms such as a powder form with a product like Natural Calm or ionic liquid form that you can add to your food and drinks. This is the most effective option for those with severe deficiency.

STEP 6

EAT COCONUT OIL

The coconut oil is the most nutrient dense part of the coconut. It will become solid at room temperature like butter. It doesn't become rancid or break down like a lot of other oils do. This is a great way to increase the healthy fats in your diet. It is also helpful in assimilation of fat soluble vitamins.

Coconut oil also has antioxidant properties and it also helps to absorb minerals. It is also a great source of Chain fatty acids (MCFAs), which have been proven to have many health benefits.

Medium Chain Fatty Acids (MCFAs). Long Chain fatty acids must be broken down before we can absorb them. Coconut oil has a high concentration of short and medium Chain fatty acids that are easy to break down and digest they are then sent to the liver for energy production.

MCFAs are good at helping to increase metabolism. They are sent straight to the liver and give the body an immediate source of energy. Most MCFAs found in coconut oil are the highly beneficial Lauric Acid.

Lauric Acid in coconut oil in combination with oregano oil has been found more effective in fighting against staph bacteria than antibiotics. Lauric acid has also been shown to help prevent certain cancers from developing. Coconut oil has over 40% Lauric acid. It is the richest source that is naturally available.

Coconut oil will be a great source in keeping good hormone health. It provides your body with the necessary building blocks it needs for hormone production, reducing inflammation, aide in weight loss, and also has antimicrobial and antibacterial properties.

STEP 7

FIXING YOUR LEPTIN

One of the master hormones is Leptin and if it is out of balance or if you are resistant to it no other hormones will balance well.

By fixing your Leptin it will help to boost fertility, improve sleep, make weight lose easier and lower inflammation.

Leptin is a master hormone in the body that controls the feelings of hunger and satiety.

Leptin is secreted by adipose (fat) tissue, so the more overweight a person is the higher his Leptin levels are going to be.

Do you have trouble sticking to a diet, crave junk foods, are overweight and want to snack especially at night? These are all signs that you could have some Leptin issues.

Leptin is known as the lookout hormone, the gatekeeper of fat metabolism, keeping track of how much energy an organism is taking in. It maintains and surveys the energy balance in your body and it regulates hunger via three pathways:

1. By counteracting the effects of neuropeptide Y, which is a potent feeding stimulant secreted by the hypothalamus and certain gut cells.
2. By counteracting the effects of anandamide, which is another feeding stimulant.
3. By promoting the production of a-MSH which is an appetite suppressant.

Leptin is also directly linked to insulin levels. Many people these days are Leptin resistant and with this come many health problems that are connected to this. Having high Leptin levels has been tied to high blood pressure, obesity, heart disease, blood sugar related problems and stroke.

High levels of Leptin with the accompanying of Leptin resistance can also decrease fertility, and age you more quickly as well as contribute to obesity.

If you are trying to lose weight or you trying to improve a health problem chances are that you have Leptin resistance. If you seem to be unable to stick to healthy changes there is a good chance that you have Leptin resistance.

Basically if you want to lose weight and make long lasting health changes you will have to fix your Leptin.

By learning how to regulate your Leptin levels you can work towards reversing Leptin resistance and its related problems but this is a complex problem that involves the endocrine system and reversing this problem will entail much more than simple calorie counting and willpower.

With most people the problem does not lie in the production of Leptin but when Leptin resistance develops it is unable to produce normal effects that will stimulate weight loss. Studies have shown that the majority of people suffering from obesity have a Leptin resistance. The Leptin resistance is understood by the body to mean starvation. So multiple mechanisms are activated to increase fat stores, rather than burn excess fat stores.
Leptin resistance also stimulates the formation of reverse T3; this blocks the effects of thyroid hormone on metabolism.

What happens is the person is eating excessive amounts of food but their body is telling them to eat more because it is starving. It is easy to understand how this cycle can contribute to weight gain.

Factors that can Contribute to Leptin Resistance

Not unlike other hormone issues Leptin resistance is a complex issue with no singular cause, but there are many factors that can have a negative impact on your Leptin levels including:

- Fructose (especially in forms like high fructose corn syrup)
- high stress levels
- exercising too much, especially if your hormones are already damaged
- overeating
- lack of sleep
- consumption of simple carbs
- high insulin levels
- grain and lectin consumption

How to Go about Fixing Leptin Resistance

This is a complex problem but it is not irreversible. Below are some non-negotiable factors that will help to improve Leptin response:

Eating no fructose, simple starches, refined foods, and sugars

After a morning walk consume a large amount of protein and healthy fats. This will help to promote satiety and will give your body the building blocks that it needs to make hormones. Try cooking scrambled eggs with some veggies add leftover meat from previous night's dinner (cook this in coconut oil).

- Be in bed by ten and optimize your sleep.
- Get outside during the day and get some skin exposed so it can absorb some vitamin D from the sun.
- Don't snack even in small amounts as this keeps your liver working and it doesn't give hormones a break. Try and set your meals so they are four hours apart then do not eat 4 hours before going to bed. You can have herbal teas without cream or sugar.

- When you are exercising only lift weights and sprint. Walk or swim if you like but don't do cardio. It is just a stress on the body. High intensity and weight lifting on the other hand give the hormone benefits of working out without the excess stress from cardio and will work great for the first few weeks. Make sure to work out in the evening not morning to help support hormone levels.
- Remove toxins from your life as these have a stress on your body.
- Eat omega-3s (fish, Chia seeds, and grass fed meats) and minimize your Omega-6 consumption (vegetable oils, grains, meats) this will help in lowering inflammation and help to support healthy Leptin levels.

Lift Heavy Weights: Extended cardio is not a good form of exercise when you are trying to fix Leptin resistance but short bursts of heavy lifting (kettle bells, lunges, squats) these can be very beneficial since they trigger a cascade of beneficial hormone reactions. Try and do a few sets (5-7) at a weight that challenges you. Make sure that you get some help if you have never trained with weights before learn how to do proper form as bad form can be harmful!

Exercising Lightly: You can make your hormone imbalance worse by participating in intense extended forms of exercise this could make the problem worse in the short term. It is more important that you get proper sleep at least during the balancing phase. Remember to focus on a relaxing form of exercise such as walking or swimming and try and stay away from running or cardio workouts.

Rebounding: Rebounding is a form of exercise that uses the forces of acceleration and deceleration that can be used to work every cell of the body in a unique way.

Rebounder (mini trampoline): When you bounce on a rebounder there are several actions that happen:
- acceleration action when you bounce upward
- there is a split-second pause at the top
- then deceleration at an increased G-force
- then you impact the rebounder
- then you repeat

The rebounding action makes use of the increased G-force from gravity with each cell in the body reacting to the acceleration and deceleration. This up and down motion is beneficial for the lymphatic system since it runs in a vertical direction within the body.

Since rebounding affects each cell in the body it can also increase cell energy and mitochondrial function. One of the greatest benefits in rebounding is to the skeletal system. This type of weight bearing exercise helps to increase bone mass. Rebounding helps to increase the weight supported by the skeletal system with the increased G-force that is created during the jumping.

Benefits of Rebounding:
- the motion of rebounding can help support the thyroid and adrenals
- can help improve muscle tone throughout the whole body
- helps to circulate oxygen throughout the body helping to increase energy
- Helps to improve effects of other exercise forms such as those that rebounded for 30 seconds between doing their weight lifting saw an increase of 25% improvement than those who did not rebound.
- It helps to improve balance by stimulating the vestibule in the middle ear
- Endurance on a cellular level is increased by stimulating the mitochondrial production which is responsible for cell energy.
- It is more effective than running without the added stress to your ankles and knees.
- Helps to increase bone mass
- Boosts lymphatic drainage and immune function

How to Get Started in Rebounding

Most sources I looked into suggested that you bounce daily for at least 15 minutes. You can break this down to 3 by 5 minute groups. When first starting just do gentle jumps with your feet still on the rebounder eventually you can build up to jumping with your feet leaving the rebounder. But it is better that you start slow and work your way up. Better to be safe than sorry.

CONCLUSION

Thank you again for purchasing this book!

I hope this book was able to help you keep your hormones balanced.

I appreciate you for taking the time out of your day or evening to read this book, and if you have an extra second, I would love to hear what you think about this book by leaving a review on Amazon. I would greatly appreciate it!

Go to http://amzn.to/1HK8rYF

If the links do not work, for whatever reason, you can simply search for the title "Hormonal Balance" on the Amazon website.

Thank you again, and I wish you nothing but the best!

Cristina Abate

HERE IS A BOOK I RECOMMEND CALLED
"FOLLOW YOUR OWN PATH"

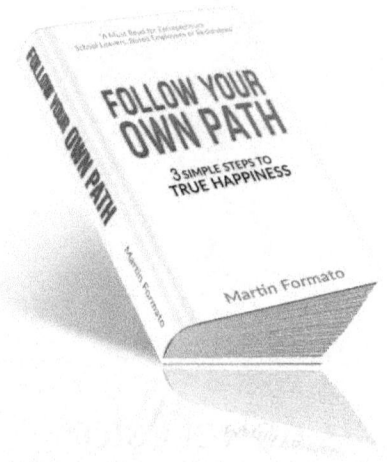

This is the coolest book I have ever read and by purchasing a copy you put another copy into the hands of someone less fortunate as the author's mission which is to inspire people to do what they love that also contributes to humanity. That is a win/win/win.

Who Is This Book For?

This book is for anyone who is hungry.

Anyone who wants more out of life.

Anyone who knows that they have more to give, share and experience.

Anyone who feels deep down, in their heart, that they are here for a reason.

It's a book for people who feel stuck, lost, depressed or even suicidal.

In particular, it's for, entrepreneurs who are struggling, school leavers who are lost, employees who are bored or in a job they hate and redundees who feel discarded.

Today, more than ever in history, people need more direction and less information.

This book will put you on the right path, YOUR PATH.

Who Is This Book NOT For?

You should not get this book until you are certain that you truly wish to change your life and you are 100 percent committed to it.

Ask yourself these 2 questions:

1. Do I want to make a change voluntarily, completely of my own choice?
2. Do I really want to change my life?

If you cannot honestly say "Yes" without hesitation to both questions, then it is better that you wait until you are serious about changing your life.

As one monk famously said "We want only warriors… victims need not apply".

Go to: http://amzn.to/2kQC9CK

If the links do not work, for whatever reason, you can simply search for the title "Follow Your Own Path" on the Amazon website.

CONTENTS FROM THE BOOK
"FOLLOW YOUR OWN PATH"

STEP 3: GIVE YOUR PASSION TO THE WORLD

Give Your Passion To The World

How Do I Start?

Planning To Live Passionately

10 Reasons Why You MUST Set Goals

Guidelines To Goal Setting

Setting Goals

Time Bound Goals

Prioritize Your Goals

Make Your Goals SMARTER

Your Life Plan On A Page

Milestones

Actions And Tasks

Goal Achievement Plan

Weekly Timetable

Things To Do Today

Living Passionately

14 Reasons Why People Don't Achieve Their Goals

Motivation And Focus

Conclusion

Resources

About The Author

Go to http://amzn.to/2kQC9CK

If the links do not work, for whatever reason, you can simply search for the title "Follow Your Own Path" on the Amazon website.

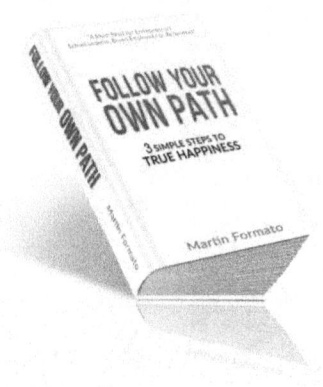

BONUS: FREE BOOK

Go to the website at www.DoingWorkThatMatters.com and enter your email address to get the FREE book "**Find Your Gift, Passion and Purpose**".

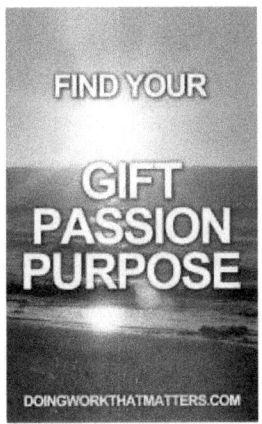

Once you register you will be sent FREE information that will further help you create a life you love.

All you have to do is enter your email address to get instant access.

This information will help you get more out of your life – to be able to reach your goals, have more motivation, be at your best, and live the life you have always dreamed of.

New resources are continually added, which you will be notified of as a subscriber. These will help you live your life to the fullest!

www.ingramcontent.com/pod-product-compliance
Lightning Source LLC
Chambersburg PA
CBHW070423190526
45169CB00003B/1381